# How to Lose Weight and Feel Great

## From A Once Overweight Person

## *by*

## *Jennifer Lukasavage*

authorHOUSE™

*1663 LIBERTY DRIVE, SUITE 200*
*BLOOMINGTON, INDIANA 47403*
*(800) 839-8640*
*WWW.AUTHORHOUSE.COM*

First published by AuthorHouse 03/09/05

ISBN: 1-4208-3355-3 (sc)

Library of Congress Control Number: 2005902238

Printed in the United States of America
Bloomington, Indiana

This book is printed on acid-free paper.

# Author's note

I am in no way a dietician or nutritionist, and what you are about to read is not medical advice.

This is written from the perspective of a formerly obese woman. I know how it feels. I know the struggle, and I know how difficult it is to overcome.

But I overcame it.

This is what worked for me.

# Table of Contents

# Introduction

My name is Jennifer Lukasavage and I wrote this book to inspire those who are overweight or what most people say are "fat". I myself was 270+ pounds and wasn't losing weight. I had just had my second child and was in a post partum depression. I have two wonderful hyper spunky boys, and a husband, and a crazy dog. It felt like the whole world was against me and I was a balloon blowing up about to pop. I could tell the way people in places I had been when I was skinny or ideal weight would stare at me. Like when your in the grocery store and your getting icecream, candy bars , and the person in back of you is like , "oh like she really needs that" but at the time I did. The food made me feel at ease. It didn't pick on me and it tasted good. But it came to

Every time I would look in the mirror all I would see is this person that sounds like me, but didn't look like the me that I was used to

Ironic how the friends that would listen to me about losing weight would lose it, but something in me just would not listen to me.

# Focus on me, myself, and I

Taking time for yourself is the most important thing you can do for yourself and for everyone else in your life. When you focus on the "me", you are saying to yourself "wow" I really care for me, to you and to everyone and that is a start. Before you can lose weight, you have to get in the state of mind that you can do it and nothing is going to stand in your way. Say to yourself, "I can do it!" "I can do it!" "I can do it!" Look in the mirror everyday and say, "I can do it!" What can you do? Is that what you are asking? You can lose the weight that you desire and no one and nothing is going to stand in your way. I know because, I was there and I did it so you can too.

Taking the time is always the problem. Making a scheduled routine and once again not letting anything get in your way. No matter if, you are sick, tired, not feeling good, too hot, too cold, and in addition, something just pursues and just continues to do it. It is hard, but you can and will do it. Focus on the "myself". By that I mean, let everyone including yourself know that you are going to take the time for yourself and let your friends and family know too. I know your saying, "Oh, well I got to do this and I got to do that.", and by the time you start, the day is over and you do not get your time in.

Taking the time for me, the you that no one knows or you might not even know that inner part of you. All parts of you need time. The you everyone sees, the one that you let everyone think you are, and the real you that if ever in your life anyone knows. Life is too short to let it go fast. The time your eating you could be exercising. The time you are talking on the phone you could be exercising. The time you are over sleeping in bed you could be exercising.

EXERCISING IS THE MOST IMPORTANT THING. EXERCISE ALL OF YOU MENTALLY, PHYSICALLY, AND SPIRITUALLY. EXERCISE, EXERCISE, EXERCISE

NOW YOU ARE PROBALLY SAYING, "OH WELL I HAVE TRIED ALL THESE OTHER BOOKS AND NOTHINGS WORKED." I KNOW, BEEN THERE, DONE THAT.

# Schedule the time

Depending on your weight depends how much time you are going to need. Example the ideal weight for a person 5 feet tall is 100 lbs. and every inch add 5 lbs. That is just an ideal of how to figure out your ideal height and weight. My height is 5'8", and I am supposed to weigh 140 lbs. on the low end and up to 160 lbs. on the high end. You have 20 lbs. to play with depending on your body frame. I have a medium to large frame so I can be on the higher end. Now the actual workout depends on you. Here are a few things that work. The ideals worked for me and I want to share them with you, so you can lose the weight too.

## *1.Buy a treadmill*

This is the best investment you can make for your health and your life. It does not matter what brand it is. Just make sure that you have a treadmill that is motorized and that it can handle your weight on it. There are many stores to pick from so I will leave that to you. Next, you schedule the time to walk on it. Make a to do list if you have to and schedule your walk in there. If you can't afford a treadmill, you can join a gym and use their treadmill or you can also walk without one, but honestly I tried that and I would cheat on time and not walk as much as I should, or as fast all the time. The treadmill gives you one speed and exact time.

A lot of gyms and exercise specialist say all you need to do is 3 times a week, but your overweight and you need to exercise everyday, not just today, but everyday. Walking is a cardiovascular exercise, so it is good for your health, heart, and it is an exercise that you can do on a daily basis and not hurt yourself. Well, you could if you do too much, too soon. Start slow and take you time. I walk everyday on my treadmill and they have timers on them so you know how much time you are spending. Here is an ideal of how to do it when you start out for the first month.

### DAY 1-7
5 minutes ce a day.
Use a slow speed 1.0.

### DAY 8-14
10 minutes twice a day.
Use speed 1.5

### DAY 15-21
15 minutes twice a day.
Use speed 2.0

### DAY 22-28
30 minutes twice a day.
Use speed 2.5

Next month increase the speed and continue to do it every month. If you can handle doing, more time and faster speeds then do it. If you at any time feel dizzy, faint, immediately slow down your speed, and if you continue to feel that way then stop and continue later as long as you get all of your time in before the day is over. That is all that matters. Right now, what I do is, I exercise once a day sometimes in the morning, afternoon, or night, and only 30 minutes for the day. I sometimes walk extra and like I said that is extra, not necessary, but nice.

## 2. *Purchase a digital scale*

You are probably saying, "This is a lot of money.", but compared to other diets, which this is not a diet, but a new way of losing weight and feeling great. I have tried many things where they make you purchase lots of foods and certain spices etc. You get the point; this is an investment for your health and life. Remember you are a very important person and deserve to get the things that will help you. I keep reminding you, because I know how it feels to feel guilty to buy things for yourself, and wind up not because you do feel guilty, but don't, you can do it, and feel proud. The scale is a fun tool to use, but use it wisely. Don't be like the old me that would jump on the scale everyday, and say, "Oh man I lost one pound." The next day comes you jump on the scale and oh boy you gained back the same pound you lost. Well here is a trick to prevent that.

## *You only weigh yourself on the scale once a week.*
## *That is right, once a week.*

The reason for weighing yourself once a week is to prevent the up, down weight gain, and lose. Your body fluctuates about 5 lbs. a week. For woman, during your menstrual period and during the time that you are having premenstrual symptoms, your body will sometimes gain up to at least 5 lbs., if not more. Some women carry water weight. Even though men do not get a physical expulsion, I still think that men also get that week a month that they get moody and need their time just like women. My husband every month around the same time gets a little bloated, moody, and irritated. Therefore, men too can have a cycle. We will call it the men cycle change of the month.

You can purchase your treadmill, scale, at any store. I got the most inexpensive, on sale ones that the stores sold. I got a digital scale with the BMI Meter (The body mass index). It tells you how fat you are, and how unhealthy you are. When I started it was a 32, which is bad, and now it is much lower. The more weight you lose, the more BMI you lose. I liked this scale compared to the others, because you punch in your height, and can save your weight for 5 days to compare. Therefore, each week you can compare from the week before and it has an arrow that tells you if your weight goes up or down and it points in that direction. It is neat and you have to try it. You can get anyone, but this is the one that I got, I do not think it matters as long as you do the exercise. The main parts of losing weight is the treadmill, the scale, and the food, which we'll get to soon enough.

# Losing the weight is all about the focusing

Remember this and keep in mind that this is not something that is gonna happen over night like surgery, but with focus and with time you will get to your goal. Give yourself time. I have lost one hundred pounds within 6 months to a year. Everyone's body is different so you could lose more weight faster or lose less weight. It's all up to you and your determination.

Now I've discussed the mental part of it. Saying to yourself, "Yes I can do it!" The physical part of it is the treadmill and walking. Now lets get to the spiritual. I have something for those who believe and don't believe. So either way I'll try to cover you.

### *For those who believe*

Tell those at your church to pray for you and your weight loss, and also pray every night for yourself.

## *For those who do not believe*

Tell yourself incantations, things like, "I can lose weight and feel great." Every day and every night. "I can lose weight and feel great." It might seem selfish at first, but everyone needs quality time for themselves and for the family.

## *Focus on the family*

Taking time for your family can be as difficult as taking time for yourself. They are both hard, but important to keep for the growth and relationships to bloom. In life we have choices and we have to continue to try to keep to the ones that make our life and living well and healthy. First you love yourself and focus on yourself, and then you focus on your family. This is the tricky part, because you have two families. You have the family that has been with you since you were born, and you have the family that you create. If you're married, you not only marry your husband , but also his family. This can be a good thing, or a bad thing. Once again if your not married, I'll give you other ideals to do with your immediate family.

We will start off with the married, dating, coupled people. Take time when you come home to have share time. Share time is when you express, how your day was, and what happened, and listen. This is the hardest part of the exercise, is the part of listening and learning not to respond, comment, or say anything until the person stops talking. This exercise releases tension, which for people who get tension like me, go straight to the refrigerator when stressed out if fighting. So stop the fighting and bickering and talk.

The next activity is to have story time with your child or children. For those who have children . If you don't have children then read one scripture a day, or read a magazine a day, read anything that stimulates your brain so it stays healthy and functional.

## *These exercises help you and your family*

Next the people who aren't married, or they are in the between stages. You can still have share time with family or friends. Everyone needs time to communicate with someone, whether it's yourself or a friend. This helps relax you and keep you emotionally kept. Keeping yourself together helps you not to over eat, or splurge, or binge.

IN ORDER TO LOSE WEIGHT AND FEEL GREAT
YOU GOTTA BELIEVE THAT YOU CAN AND WILL
DO IT.
IT'S A STATE OF MIND.

Keep your family and friends involved in what you're doing and how your doing with what you are doing. If that makes any sense. I'm telling you to involve your family, friends, and neighbors, and anyone. By letting everyone know that you're trying to lose weight. Sometimes when you're losing weight, you don't see what everyone else sees. You get encouragement, support systems, help, and make new friends.

For those who don't have friends or family. You can join a group through your school, church, or your local borough or township. There are lots of programs out there. They all are great programs. If you can't afford them, then look in your local town newspaper and there are free groups you can attend.

Basically, you need support, you need support and self esteem from yourself and others to get you through this hard time. It is hard. You see all these skinny people and say, "Ooooh laaaalaaaaaaa, that could be me." Then you get depressed and eat, and don't exercise.

STOP STOP STOP STOP STOP STOP STOP!!!

DON'T BE SO HARD ON YOURSELF. YOU CAN DO IT. IT'S JUST GONNA TAKE TIME AND SUPPORT, AND A LITTLE COOPERATION.

Sometimes you can get your friends and family to join in with you on your journey of losing weight. I got my mom to get a treadmill, and a scale, and now she is losing weight and feeling great too. I also got my friends to join in on losing weight.

It's all about believing you can lose the weight and actually losing the weight. The first few months it's hard, because you got to train your mind and body to do the job you have in store for it. When your mind, and body are joined together and cooperating with each other it makes your journey an easy one. Remember to try to get everyone involved in this journey with you and to keep it real.

YOU CAN AND WILL LOSE WEIGHT
AND FEEL GREAT
YOU CAN AND WILL LOSE WEIGHT
AND FEEL GREAT

# Focus on the positive

You also have to think positive and positive will come to you. I use this saying all the time.

## THINK POSITIVE AND POSITIVE WILL COME TO YOU

Example with myself, when I started saying, "I can lose weight and feel great." I started to lose the weight.

## THINK NEGATIVE AND NEGATIVE WILL COME TO YOU

Example with myself, when I started saying, "I'm fat, I'm pathetic, I'm a blimptoid, I'm a chubby bubby cow." I started to believe it and get in a depressed state of mind, which made me over eat and gain weight.

Your next step is to think positive, so that you start to act positive, think positive, look positive, and everyone, including you knows that you will make it and achieve your goals.

I know sometimes in life, it is hard when you have a full-time job, you have work demands, and you are a homemaker, or have a part-time job. Work demands can be harder sometimes than your family. You start to ignore your family for your job and both stress you out. Stress can cause you despair and anguish, and hurt you mentally. Just use this saying repeatedly until it makes you sick and you use it.

## THINK POSITIVE AND POSITIVE WILL COME TO YOU

## THINK POSITIVE AND POSITIVE WILL COME TO YOU

Think of yourself as a trophy, which brings you joy. It needs sparkling, and cleaning. You spend attention looking at it, and holding it. You even share the time and talk explaining how you achieved it. Think of yourself the same way. I always say, "whatever". If you do not do it for yourself, who will. You have to let your mind and will power gets over the urges and craves for food, or whatever your addition is. Usually, the food addition makes you gain the weight.

Anyone can take my advice and use it, or you read this and say, "Of all the nerve." The truth is you have to take the time. The time to know, believe that you can and will lose the weight and feel great. TAKE IT FROM A ONCE FAT PERSON. I know how it is to be put down and humiliated. It hurts and puts your self-esteem in a hole. You feel like your falling and you cannot get up or out of it, but you just want to. The only way that you can is by ignoring them, and saying to yourself, "I can lose the weight and feel great." Thinking positive takes time and is sometimes the hardest thing to achieve.

I sometimes read the bible and cannot believe how someone could love strangers and people and die for their sins. I know I could not do it, but at least someone did it for me.

FOR GOD SO LOVED THE WORLD THAT HE GAVE HIS ONLY BEGOTTON SON THAT WHOSOEVER BELIEVETH IN HIM SHALL NOT PERISH BUT HAVE EVERLASTING LIFE.
John 3:16

For those who believe, just this phrase should help you think positive. Out of respect for those who do not believe, you can think of it like this. The wind is there, you do not always see it, or feel it, but you know that it is there. Grass, it grows sometimes with help and sometimes by itself. We all need help sometimes and by thinking positive, it gives you a head start to getting the job done. Losing weight to some people is by surgery, others by pills, drugs, or whatever floats their boat. I am trying to help you learn the techniques that I am using. So that you can live a long and healthy life. The grass is not always greener on the other side. You look at people, get jealous, and say, "That could be me." Guess what? That could be you with some time, perseverance, and dedication.

I CAN DO ALL THINGS THRU CHRIST WHO
STRENGHTHENS ME.

The next thing is getting a goal and sticking to it no matter how hard it seems to be to achieve. Once you set it, do not let go no matter what. You can and will do it. You will lose the weight and feel great.

# Focus on the goal

The goal is the amount of weight that you want to lose. Do not be hard on yourself, make an outrageous number, and think that it is going to happen overnight. Unless you have surgery, then it is not. Set a realistic goal. It can be a high number, but keep in mind that it will take some time and energy. It will take some determination from you to meet this goal. 100 pounds is going to take you at least 6mths.-one year to do, but your doing it a healthy and safe way. Losing too much weight too soon can hurt you. Setting your goal for how much time you are going to spend on your treadmill.

## GOAL #1
Make a scheduled time to exercise.

## GOAL#2
Make a reasonable weight desire.

## GOAL#3
Focus! Focus! Focus!

After making your three important goals, then you must do it. Do not make excuses, or let anything stand in your way. You are a strong person that can do anything once you put your mind to it. If I can do it, anyone can do it. I was a hopeless case I thought and went from size 20 down to a size 10. When I look at my old pants, I cannot believe how big I was. If I can go down 100lbs., so can you. It does take a while, but with strength and endurance, you too can do it. I still exercise and continue to maintain and set my goals and am still losing weight and feeling great. That is the whole point of this, is to help people lose naturally, safe, and effectively. Everyone that has taken my advice in doing this has lost the weight. You too can lose the weight.

Make your goals apart of your life, as well as your family and friends. When you have people involved in your life with your goals and focus, sometimes it helps you stay on track. Your friends can help you when you are supposed to be exercising and your reaching for your cookies and doughnuts. Your friend will say, "No.No.No.Don't do it." That will help you keep on goal. Support systems help maintain and balance you. Just as you balance, your checkbook or else you do not know how much money you have. Do the same for your life. You have to balance and maintain it so you stay healthy and fit. If you do not you will be six feet under too soon. Do not let the fear stop you from doing what you want to.

When you make goals to lose weight, it becomes a reality, because you intend to keep the goals. It is just like making a list. When you make a shopping list, you buy everything on that list, and if the thing that you want is not, there you replace it with something else. It is the same with losing the weight. You make the goal to lose the weight and lose the weight. It is not just physical, but is emotional, mental. Your whole self has to be involved in this process.

Make your goals the same as a list. Do not give yourself too many goals to discourage yourself, but make a realistic amount. Make three goals. Just like on New Years Eve, You make a New Years solution. Do the same thing with your goals. Make it happen. You are the potter with the clay. You can mold it and make it any shape, size, that you want. Make your goals. Getting your friends and family involved. Your significant other also can get involved in helping you towards your goals.

KEEP IN MIND NOT TO ALLOW YOUR FRIENDS, FAMILY, AND SIGNIFICANT OTHER TO MAKE YOUR GOALS. THE GOALS HAVE TO BE YOURS AND ONLY YOURS. FOR THEN YOU WILL ACHIEVE THEM.

When you do things for other people you will eventually resent them, and over eat or splurge or just not do what you want to out of resentment. Make sure that you do it for yourself, because I have been there too. You want to make someone else happy that you hurt yourself in the process of helping them get towards their goals and never finish your own. It is not being selfish to take care of yourself and to love yourself, and respect yourself enough to make these goals happen. You are a very important person and you deserve the best. Do not let anyone tell you different.

MAKE YOUR GOALS, KEEP THEM, DO THEM, AND
LOVE THEM.

MAKE YOUR GOALS, KEEP THEM, DO THEM, AND
LOVE THEM.

Love yourself enough to do the things that will help you get there. You too can succeed, just like the others that have done it and are doing it. You too can be that one that says to yourself, "I did it and I'm happy I made the goal to lose the weight and feel great and that I read this book and took the time and effort to do it."

# Focus on the food

This is going to get into the part you all have been waiting for. The part where you say, "Oh I can or can't do it." I know you can though. I will discuss what you can eat, and should not eat. Keep in mind that everyone's body is different so you can change a few things to your satisfaction. For breakfast, you want a big well maintenance diet. Not a diet, but a meal plan. A routine breakfast that will not make you gain, but keep you filled and happy until lunch and dinner. Here are a few ideas to use.

# Let's get to eating!

## *Breakfast*

#1
One cup of raisin bran, or granola.
Any brand is ok.

One cup of milk
Try to use 2% and lower if possible.

One cup of orange juice.
Any brand is ok.  I use the low acid kind so you can drink
it everyday and not get a stomachache.
#2

One cup of low carb yogurt.
It tastes like regular yogurt, just not all the fat or carbs.

One banana.

One cup of orange juice.


#3

One 16oz.of coffee or tea.

One breakfast bar.

## *Lunch*

#1

One cup of yogurt.
Any brand is ok.

One cup of grapes.
Any kind will be fine.

One apple
Any kind, I love granny smith

One cup of iced tea or soda
Any brand.

#2

Two cups of salad.
Any brand, kind or pre-made.

Italian salad dressing.
Any brand is ok.

One cup of iced tea or soda.
Try to drink light colored soda.

One cup of carrots, half of a cup of tomatoes.
Get the baby carrots and the grape tomatoes.

### #3

One 12 inch or smaller.
Turkey or chicken hoagie.
Lettuce, tomatoes, onions.
Lite, if you use mayo, or oil.
Use mustard.
Use salt, pepper, oregano.
Sweet peppers, pickles.

One cup of iced tea or soda.

## Dinner

### #1

Use one box of hamburger, tuna, or chicken box meals.
Only eat two bowls if eating alone.
Save the rest for the next night.

Broccoli.
Some kind of vegetable.

One cup of iced tea or soda.
As much of it as you want.

### #2

One steak.

One bowl of rice and beans.

Vegetables.
Drink.

#3

Pizza with veggies on it.
Spinach, mushrooms.
Four slices the most.

Drink.

## Snack

#1

One bag of popcorn.
Use lite, if you use butter.

One bottled water.

#2

One cup of pretzels.

One bottled water.

#3

One banana or piece of fruit.

One bottled water.

## YOU WANT TO EAT SIX TIMES A DAY

## BREAKFAST, SNACK, LUNCH, SNACK, DINNER, SNACK

Your vitamins are also important. Use daily, take once a day. Any brand is good. Use calcium pills, if you are not getting enough milk. When you are sick, take one vitamin C 500mg. and one vitamin E 500mg. drink your minimum of eight glasses of water a day. Drink bottled water, and then you know that you are drinking enough water. When you walk on your treadmill, you will get thirsty, so drink water. Buy the water bottles so you know that you are drinking the right amount of water and so you drink it. Any brand is ok. When you are exercising, have four bottles of 16oz. with you. Then you have your eight glasses of water. Every 5 minutes, drink half of one of the bottles. By 30 minutes, all will be gone.

All of this is new to you so eating two bowls of something instead of four will be hard and take time to where your stomach will feel full with just two bowls. Drinking the water with the exercise helps you to get the water that you are body needs and your eight glasses in. Exercise and proper eating is important. If you continue to eat too much, you will not gain or lose any weight. If for a week you over eat, try to continue to do the exercise. Do not get discouraged; it is just that you are used to over-eating. Think positive and lose the weight the next week.

Do not give up or stop. Sometimes the body goes in cycles where it will not lose weight and that is ok. Then the next week, it will seem like you lost much more than you are supposed to. That is normal and can be expected. Focus on maintaining proper eating and proportions. Use measuring cups and measuring spoons until it becomes habit. With time, you will lose the weight and feel great.

# Focus on reality check

HERE IS SOMETHING I WROTE WHEN I WAS
GRADUATING CLASS OF 95.

LIFE! NATURE!!

How precious it is and we just use it. Things that are small become big and tall or large. Times go by and we do not appreciate things until it is too late. We just use it up and allow things to continue, since it is a non-stop essence of life. A clock is there, but actually is only a figment of imagination. No one can ever really know what time is now or then. People can be small, tall, skinny, medium, large, big, chunky, huge, etc. However, all are united by the reality of life. People can only last so long on a trip or fantasy, but one thing never changes and that is the cycle. It grows and continues until who knows? Only one holds that key and is not going to give it free to anyone. Who should judge this simple fact of life? Life to some means a new creation, a new baby, animal, etc. Life and its whole meaning of everything. If life did not exist neither would anyone, or at that anything. Do not give up on life until you have given your all into life. If you have ever just relaxed and here is an example: Just sit down by a tree or anywhere and just think about the simple little things such as:
> 1. Leaves growing.
> 2. Hair growing, at that anything growing.

Nature seems to bring calm, peace, and a tender eye to all who can or are willing to listen, look, and appreciate all that it tries to tell or show us. Life is there for those who do and do not believe. See you had to believe in order for it to grow once you planted a plant. Why do people not believe in Jesus when he actually already was here and yet he spoke, showed, proved himself, but still people do not believe he was the chosen one? God's son. That is all apart of human nature. Allows people to be, show, and do whatever they want. It might not always be right or even planned, but they still can do it. Due to society the group of people who majorize us, they make the government, the ruler over all and that freedom in life is gone to an extent.

See no matter what anyone says, you can always do whatever, but now there are expectations of punishment, some kind of result is or will take place. Back to the main point, LIFE. Life is the basis of all creatures, all things, all of everything. Nature on the other hand, is a part of life giving reasoning and aspects of good parts of life, also it shows downfall when not taken care of, treated, or helped. In actual reality, this pertains to the main fact, all know they are destined to help, but choose at one time or another not to, but later on realize how just them actually brought a downfall on all, all of life. Whether or not you realize it or not we all are life, life in nature. Nature in life.

Meaning, we as people are a society, a group, large populated one, where we make things to come or go. We affect all, but do not seem to realize it until it is too late. Almost anything, even the simplest looking substance such as a flower, it may look simple, easy to take down, but it took in all, many things in life to become the actual flower it became.

Everything, everyone has its difficulties. Just like the rose dies, so must people and animal, or anything living. All live in the life cycle. Life to all has different ideas, meanings. My idea is only a standard, or should I say a realist ideal, but who should say that. For then I could be trying to change the actual, factual cycle of life. I would not want to do that for then I would get the consequences for messing with life.

Life to all as once say before in this essay means different things to all. To some, Life means all science, some faith, some this, and some that. I could continue on everything everyone else has said or spoken on life, but instead I chose to give you my choice of meanings.

Life is beautiful. Nature is beautiful. Both are aspects of life. Life in overall is the one thing all need to survive to live. To live means to use life. I am trying to express how life in nature, which really is life, is beautiful if one or people choose to take the time to look at it. Try it.

1. Just, close your eyes and allow yourself to meditate on life. It is beautiful. Just listen bump, bump,—bump, bump-bump, bump, the sound of a heartbeat. This process expresses how life is so complicated, and yet, easy to end.

2. Open and close your hand. Eyes open or closed, it does not matter. This is another process so easy to do, but really takes a lot of energy to do.

3. Open and close your mouth and breathe in, and breathe out. You have now experienced life from two aspects of life.

    A. The process of breathing and movement.

    B. Breathing using plants $CO_2$ and the breathing process.

4. Smell, now that is another process.

I could go on and on with processes of just the person, human beings, but that's just a point getting a crossed to all. Life is a part of all, everything alone. Life is the essential over all, also expresses how nature in life helps humans. Just the few examples of processes express the complexity of oneself, one's state of mind. The major point I am trying to get to you all is life. Live for life, for life will outlive all life, but would like people to appreciate it. For it will continue throughout all people, things, and continue.

Once you have lost life, its then past and all that could have been yours is lost. Do not allow this life process to get one self down, but instead live for life, because after all life lives for you. One more example of focusing on reality is this:

1. Exercise.
2. Eat well-balanced meals.
3. Lose weight and feel great.
4.

### *Keep things in threes to remember*

# Here's a little poem to end my book about a little birdie

Way up yonder up on those hills is trees and one of those trees is special. For it has life upon it, it contains a nest with hatched birds upon it. The birds stay and chirp while the mother flies in to look for food to feed the babies. The mother comes upon a worm and brings it back to the nest. Afterwards it is time for them to learn how to fly for seasons a changin' and they will die from the cold breeze a blowin' in from the winds. The season is winter. As the babies try desperately to learn to fly, they finally learn and are ready for the flight. They are up and a flyin'. They finally make it to the south and learn the importance of flyin'.

I wrote this poem from 12th grade. This is just to get you started and to believe in yourself and just let go and fly like the birdies and do it. You can fly and be free and take care of yourself. Love yourself enough to do the necessary things to help yourself out of whatever is holding you back from doing what you must do. You can and will lose weight and feel great. Instead of making exercise a chore, make it a routine and enjoy knowing that if it can work for me, then it can work for you.

# Overview

1. Take time for me, myself, and I.
2. Take the time for the family.
3. Take the time to be positive.
4. Take the time to make the goal.
5. Take the time to eat food.
6. Take the time to relax.
7. Exercise and lose weight and feel great.

You never know what life is going to throw you, so keep your hands up and catch it. You do not know when it is your last day, so live it. You never know anything, but you can know that you can and will do these simple things and lose the weight and feel great. What do you have to lose? If anything, you learn how to exercise, and learn how to take time for you, and everything around you.

YOU CAN DO THIS.
YOU CAN DO THIS.
YOU CAN DO THIS.

# Conclusion

I really want to share with you all what worked for me, and hopefully will work for you. I have always wanted to write a book and was always too tired to do anything. Being overweight consumed me mentally, physically, and spiritually. Mentally, just looking at myself I had no desire to do anything, but live and pay bills and taxes. Physically, I just wanted to, but could not because of being too tired, and being overweight causes extra heat and you lose a lot of energy. Spiritually, depressed, because why did this happen to me? Then I thought about it one day and said,

"Something has got to change!", and I did it. I let the little light in my head click. I chose to do whatever it would take to do it until I got what I achieved for, no matter what. I chose to lose weight and feel great. Keep in mind that it will not happen overnight, but it will happen. It honestly took me about 6mths.-one year to achieve my goal. For some it could be faster, for some it could take longer. The point of my book is to share with those who are overweight, or not happy with their current weight to lose it, and do it in a safe and natural way. There are no drugs, no eating food that you do not like, or starving yourself. Just doing what you enjoy and taking the extra time to measure and proportion and still enjoy the foods you love and adore.

I love food and understand how it can be for someone to say, "Oh you can't have this, and you can't have that." Therefore, that is why I wrote this book. Many people will look at the fact that it took me 6mths. - Year, but the only thing that is going to work overnight is surgery. The truth is that usually when you are overweight that you cannot have surgery, or should not because of complications due to the weight. Usually you blood pressure gets higher with the more weight you have too. Many things can happen because of being overweight. Please for your sake just try it. I am sure if you are like me, that you have probably tried it all. You just have to get in the state of mind that no matter what you are and will lose the weight if it takes forever and then gradually and steady, it happens. You do not start to notice it until one day your friend or associate at work asks you what you are doing. What are you doing? That is what they will say and hopefully you will say, "I'm losing weight and feeling great." I read this book by a new author who once was overweight, I tried what worked for her, and it worked for me too. Let us do it together and see how fast it works for us. Let us help each other keep the courage and strength to complete this task, goal of losing the weight. I know that it is achievable, because I did it. I wrote this in hope that others too can achieve the same goals and dreams as me. When you put your mind to something, nothing is impossible.

## ALL THINGS ARE POSSIBLE THRU CHRIST WHO STRENGHTENS ME.

This is an important verse. You can do it and achieve your goal. You can lose the weight. You can eat the food you like, or the food I like. You can still eat sweets. I love cookies. In the beginning, lower the intake, but do not stop all together. If you can do the cold turkey method, then do it. However, if you are like me and a whole lot of people who cannot do that then take your time and work gradually to that point. It is not going to happen in one day, but it will happen. I hope and pray that you will be as successful as I was and am continuing on my process. If I can do it, then you can and will do it too.

Love yourself enough to take the time to do this. You can and will lose the weight and feel great. You will achieve your goal, no matter how long it takes. Do not get discouraged when you are right around the corner from your goal weight and all of a sudden, you stay at the same weight for a few weeks. That is normal and a pain in the butt. Sometimes when you get to this point, you have to do a little more sometimes. Everybody is different so keep that in mind. You just have to believe in yourself that you can do it, and you will not let anyone or anything stand in your way.

YOU CAN LOSE WEIGHT AND FEEL GREAT.
YOU CAN LOSE WEIGHT AND FEEL GREAT.
YOU CAN LOSE WEIGHT AND FEEL GREAT.

Do not be scared to get your family and friends involved in this process with you. I am a homemaker, all the food is there, and sometimes you cannot stop. I know, been there, done that. When you are a homemaker sometimes, you do not have many friends and can tend to get depressed. It is important for the ones you do have, to know what you are attempting to do. I only have one best friend and it helps. Also, let your spouse: husband or wife, or even your partner know so they can help you on your quest, journey, or mission, whatever you must say to do it.

## KEEPING IT REAL ABOUT ME AND MY ACHIEVEMENTS

## I TRY TO KEEP AN OPEN MIND TO ALL WHO READ THIS BOOK. IF I HAVE OFFENDED YOU, I APOLIGIZE, BUT THAT IS JUST ME AN OVERTALKATIVE, BLUNT TALKING AND WRITING PERSON.

Please remember that I once was overweight, obese for my height and weight proportion. I had a high body mass index. I know how it feels to look in the mirror and sometimes cry or get upset with what you see. I know how it feels to get depressed, oversleep, and overeat. I have been there, done that. I do know. If I can do it, then you too can do it.

I set my goal right after I had my second son to lose the weight. That would be June, 2003. I was about 270-300lbs. When you get big, you stop going on the scale as much. My goal for myself was to lose 100lbs., possibly more. I have done this. I was a size 20, and now am a size 10. I have gone done ½ of my size. I bought the treadmill around Oct. or Nov. and did not use it regularly. It took me the New Year's resolution of losing weight or just the desire to do it. I started exercising everyday starting Jan.1ˢᵗ 2004. That is when I saw a difference. My friends or associates did not notice until about March or April, which is only 3-4 months.

Every month I would lose one pant size. I started at 20.

| | |
|---|---|
| JAN 04 | 18-20 |
| FEB 04 | 16-18 |
| MARCH 04 | 14-16 |
| APRIL 04 | 12-14 |
| MAY 04 | 10-12 |
| JUNE 04 | 9-10 |

If someone tells you it is going to happen overnight, it is definitely a lie. Even with surgery, it takes a few months. With time and effort, you can achieve your goals. If you have tried it, all like me, then give this a shot. What do you have to lose, but the weight? I know with the time and goal, you too can achieve your goal like. For some you could lose more or less weight. No one gains or loses the same way. Remember you are a unique individual and you will lose the weight your body loses weight. Overall, you will lose the weight and feel great. You can and will do it. It is all about getting to that point where you just cannot take it anymore and act on those feelings. Take the initiative to meet your goal.

## FOR ALL OF YOU WHO HAVE ENJOYED THIS BOOK AND THOSE WHO HAVE NOT.

I hope that this works for you just like it has for me. I hope that you stick to the goal and make it happen. I hope that with the help from yourself, friends, and family you get the support that you need. I hope that you make your dream come true. I hope that you lose the weight and feel great. Sorry to those of you who do not like this, this is my first book. Thanks to all of you who have helped and supported me. At that note, I will say goodbye.

PLEASE DO NOT FORGET TO TELL EVERYONE ABOUT THIS BOOK, MAKE IT LIKE A CHAIN LETTER. NEVERTHELESS, INSTEAD IT WILL BE ONE OF THE FIRST CHAIN BOOKS. YOU HAVE TO TELL ONE PERSON ABOUT THIS BOOK.

KEEP A LOOK OUT FOR MY NEXT BOOK: BOOK #2 SKINCARE, MAKE-UP FOR THE NEW YOU

# Meal
# Charts
# &
# Tips For
# Healthy Eating

Cut or tear these pages out for easy reference!

| MONDAY | TUESDAY | WEDNESDAY | THURSDAY | FRIDAY |
|--------|---------|-----------|----------|--------|
| **BREAKFAST** | **BREAKFAST** | **BREAKFAST** | **BREAKFAST** | **BREAKFAST** |
| ONE CUP OF RAISIN BRAN ANY BRAND | ONE CUP OF YOGURT ANY BRAND | ONE CUP OF COFFEE OR TEA | ONE CUP OF GRANOLA ANY FLAVOR | ONE CUP OF YOGURT ANY BRAND |
| ONE CUP OF MILK 2% OR LESS | ONE BANANA | ONE BREAKFAST BAR | ONE CUP OF MILK 2% OR LESS | ONE CUP OF FRUIT DRINK |
| ONE CUP OF ORANGE JUICE | ONE CUP OF ORANGE JUICE | | ONE CUP OF ORANGE JUICE | |

| SATURDAY | SUNDAY |
|---|---|
| **BREAKFAST** | **BREAKFAST** |
| ONE DOUGHNUT | ONE CUP OF CEREAL |
| ONE CUP OF COFFEE OR TEA | ONE CUP OF MILK 2% OR LESS |
| | ONE CUP OF ORANGE JUICE |

*Jennifer Lukasavage*

| MONDAY LUNCH | TUESDAY LUNCH | WEDNESDAY LUNCH | THURSDAY LUNCH | FRIDAY LUNCH |
|---|---|---|---|---|
| ONE CUP OF YOGURT ANY BRAND | TWO CUPS OF SALAD ANY BRAND | ONE TURKEY HOAGIE | ONE CAN OF CHICKEN SOUP ANY BRAND | ONE CHICKEN HOAGIE |
| ONE CUP OF FRUIT EX. GRAPES | ITALIAN DRESSING | LETTUCE TOMATOES ONIONS | ONE CUP OF SALAD ANY BRAND | LETTUCE TOMATOES ONIONS |
| ONE APPLE | ONE CUP OF BABY PEELED CARROTS | LITE ON MAYO AND OIL MUSTARD | ITALIAN DRESSING | LITE ON MAYO AND OIL MUSTARD |
| ONE CUP OF TEA OR SODA OR WATER | ONE CUP OF GRAPE TOMATOES | USE SPICES, SALT PEPPER OREGANO | HALF CUP OF BABY PEELED CARROTS | USE SPICES, SALT, PEPPER OREGANO |
| | | SWEET PEPPERS PICKLES | HALF CUP OF GRAPE TOMATOES | SWEET PEPPERS PICKLES |
| | ONE CUP OF TEA OR SODA OR WATER | ONE CUP OF TEA OR SODA OR WATER | ONE CUP OF TEA OR SODA OR WATER | ONE CUP OF TEA OR SODA OR WATER |

| SATURDAY | | SUNDAY | |
| --- | --- | --- | --- |
| LUNCH | | LUNCH | |
| PEANUT BUTTER AND JELLY ANY BRAND | | ONE BEAN BURRITO | |
| ONE CARROT OR CELERY | | ONE APPLE OR ORANGE | |
| ONE CUP OF TEA OR SODA OR WATER | | ONE CUP OF TEA OR SODA OR WATER | |

| MONDAY | TUESDAY | WEDNESDAY | THURSDAY | FRIDAY |
|--------|---------|-----------|----------|--------|
| **DINNER** | **DINNER** | **DINNER** | **DINNER** | **DINNER** |
| TWO BOWLS OF HAMBURGER BOXED MEALS | ONE SLICE OF STEAK | TWO BOWLS OF TUNA BOXED MEALS | TWO BOWLS OF CHICKEN BOXED MEALS | 2-4 SLICES OF PIZZA |
| ONE CUP OF BROCCOLLI SPICES OR CHEESE | ONE BOWL OF RICE AND BEANS | ONE CUP OF PEAS OR MIXED VEGGIES | ONE CUP OF MIXED VEGGIES | PUT VEGGIES ON IT LIKE SPINACH BROCCOLLI |
| ONE CUP OF TEA OR WATER | ONE CUP OF MIXED VEGGIES | ONE CUP OF TEA OR WATER | ONE CUP OF TEA OR WATER | ONE CUP OF TEA OR WATER |
| | ONE CUP OF TEA OR WATER | | | |

| SATURDAY | SUNDAY |
|----------|--------|
| **DINNER** | **DINNER** |
| ONE CUP OF FRUIT | ONE SLICE OF TURKEY OR CHICKEN SAUSAGE |
| ONE CUP OF VEGGIES | ONE CUP OF VEGGIES |
| ONE CUP OF TEA OR WATER | ONE CUP OF TEA OR WATER |

| MONDAY | TUESDAY | WEDNESDAY | THURSDAY | FRIDAY |
|--------|---------|-----------|----------|--------|
| **SNACK** | **SNACK** | **SNACK** | **SNACK** | **SNACK** |
| YOGURT ANY BRAND ONE CUP | PRETZELS ONE CUP | ONE BREAKFAST BAR | FRUIT ONE APPLE | ONE BAG OF MICROWAVE POPCORN |
| WATER | WATER | WATER | WATER | WATER |

| | SATURDAY | | | | SUNDAY | |
|---|---|---|---|---|---|---|
| | **SNACK** | ONE CUP OF LOW FAT ICECREAM | WATER | | **SNACK** | 2 OATMEAL COOKIES | WATER |

# Smoothie Recipe

INGREDIENTS:
Orange juice
Banana
Ice

Use a blender or smoothie machine.
I use a blender and put one cup of orange juice.
One banana.
Use seven ice cubes to make it cold.
Then blend it and enjoy.

YOU CAN ADD MANY OTHER GOODIES TO THIS:
3 Strawberries          3 Pineapple slices
3 Blueberries          3 Apple slices
Three Raspberries

THE LIST COULD GO ON EVEN ADDING VEGGIES:
FOR THOSE WHO DO LIKE VEGGIES THIS IS
GREAT FOR YOU:
Three baby all ready peeled carrots

# Tips for healthy eating

You can eat the Tuesday salad meal everyday, because it is very healthy and well balanced. I usually eat this everyday. For those who get bored there are different options.

Try not to eat pork, pork is not healthy or clean for you. It causes a lot of weight gain, and oils in your body, which can also cause skin problems, like acne.

Try to eat before 6o'clock at night.  Eat at certain times to prevent overeating.

Get on a routine so your body gets used to it..

YOU WANT TO EAT SIX TIMES A DAY

| BREAKFAST | 6 AM |
|-----------|------|
| SNACK | 9 AM |
| LUNCH | 12 PM |
| SNACK | 3 PM |
| DINNER | 6 PM |
| SNACK | 9 PM |

## *Carbs*

You do not want to eat carbs all day either.  What are carbs?  They are things like pasta, and bread.  So try to moderate how much of that you consume.  They also came out with low carb yogurts, which really taste good.  They have all kind of flavors. I have tasted a lot of them and they are good.  For bread, instead of eating regular white bread, eat wheat or 12 grain, when eating sandwiches. In addition, for pasta they have vegetable spinach, garden pasta, which tastes the same, but has less carbs.  You want to decrease your pasta, bread, and increase your veggies.  Just like all the other books out there.  You must eat and keeping the food pyramid in check.

# Food Pyramid

### Veggies
Buy the mixed veggie cans or raw is fine.

### Fruit
Buy fresh, the cans have too much sugar juice.

### Meats
Buy only turkey, chicken, beef, fish, and no pork.

### Dairy
Use less percentage, instead of whole use 2%

## *Sweets*

For those of you who love sweets and cannot get rid of them, but now you enjoy them on the weekends, instead of everyday. This is good for you until you can put a quit to the sweets all together. I am still working on it too.

If you drink soda, then try to drink light colored sodas. Drink these until you can try and not drink soda at all. Just try to drink less each day. Soda causes stomach problems for some and the carbonation can sometimes cause you to gain more weight and faster. They also make lite, sodas, which you can try.

## *Junk Food*

Try to eat the junk food only on the weekends. You can do this until you can let go all together. It takes a lot of work to let go. I am still working on it. You can lose the weight and feel great with a lot of time and effort. This is achievable. You can and will do it. Everyday remind yourself of the goal and even when you get depressed and eat the whole container of ice cream and the whipped cream, you still can make it. Yes, I am talking about things I have done. You can always switch things around, but if you eat more of something that you should not, then you should make it up on the treadmill, or park.

Remember everyday on the treadmill. No, slack whatever. Walking at a school or park is extra walking and losing weight and toning. Make it your routine of walking on the treadmill, everyday. Yes, everyday. If I can do it, I know that anyone can do it.

# About the Author

Jennifer Lukasavage lives in a family town Bridgeport, Pennsylvania where her and her husband raise their two sons, a dog, two turtles, two hermit crabs, and a goldfish. She is a homemaker who was once overweight and wrote a book about how she lost weight. This is her 1st book she has written, and is trying to write a second book. She wrote this book with faith that others too would lose the weight and feel great with her.